MY FIRST
Number Tracing
WORKBOOK

MY FIRST Number Tracing WORKBOOK

Practice Pen Control *with* Numbers

Rachael Smith

ROCKRIDGE PRESS

Series Designer: Stephanie Mautone
Interior and Cover Designer: Stephanie Mautone
Art Producer: Tom Hood
Editor: Eliza Kirby
Production Editor: Andrew Yackira
Production Manager: Jose Olivera

Cover and interior photography © Shutterstock, 2021
Author photograph courtesy Jaime Healy

ISBN: Print 978-1-64876-402-8
R0

This book belongs to:

_____

For the Parents

If you are reading this, you are the proud parent of a preschooler who is learning numbers and letters. This book will help your child learn to read, write, and count numbers while teaching them how to hold and use a pen. The fun and engaging activities in each section are designed for children from three to five years old. We will begin with tracing exercises that develop and strengthen pen control. Your little one will practice forming a variety of line types, starting with straight lines and progressing to zigzags and curves. This will help them develop the skills needed to form numbers.

The second section will gradually introduce the numbers 0 to 20. On each page there are tracing outlines of the numeral and the number word. There is also space to copy the numbers freehand without pre-drawn lines. Review activities throughout this section will reinforce the skills your child has learned and invite them to start counting.

Learning to write and comprehend numbers creates a strong foundation to build future math knowledge. Basic number sense is needed for many future math tasks, as well as current ones. Little ones enjoy counting their toys and treats. They'll notice if they get more cookies than someone else and knowing numbers will help them learn to share. Building their understanding of numbers will open the door for effectively communicating in their everyday life as they prepare for school. Whether your child is just beginning to learn to write, or is perfecting their skills, we hope that this book is an enjoyable learning tool.

Prewriting Activities

●▲■▼▽●◗◖●▲■▼▽●◗◖●▲■▼▽●◗◖●▲■

DIRECTIONS

In this section, your little writer will complete tracing activities while developing the fine motor skills needed to write numbers and letters independently. They will copy different types of lines, from straight to jagged to curvy. These deliberate motions will help them improve their pen control. The skills they develop in this prewriting section will benefit them as they move on to tracing numbers in the next section of the book.

These activities were designed with preschoolers in mind, and should spark conversations about colors, shapes, weather, and animals. As your little one traces and colors, keep them engaged with meaningful conversation that explores these topics.

Remember, controlling a pen can be difficult at first. Praise your child as they practice, and gently encourage them to hold the writing utensil correctly if they struggle. When children are beginning to write, a thick and chunky writing utensil, like a crayon or thick pencil, can be easier for them to control. These positive experiences will boost their confidence and motivate them to continue building these important skills that they will use throughout their life.

Happy writing!

Trace the numbers.

0 1 2 3

4 5 6 7

8 9 10

11 12 13

14 15

16 17 18

19 20

Trace the dotted lines to match each baby animal to its mother.

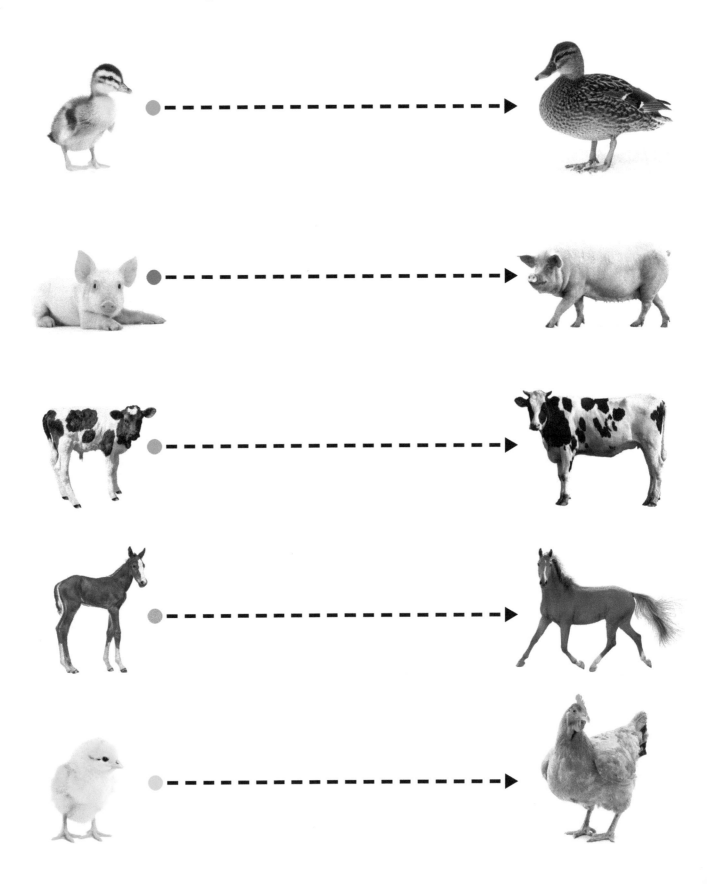

It's raining, it's pouring! Trace the dotted lines to complete the picture.

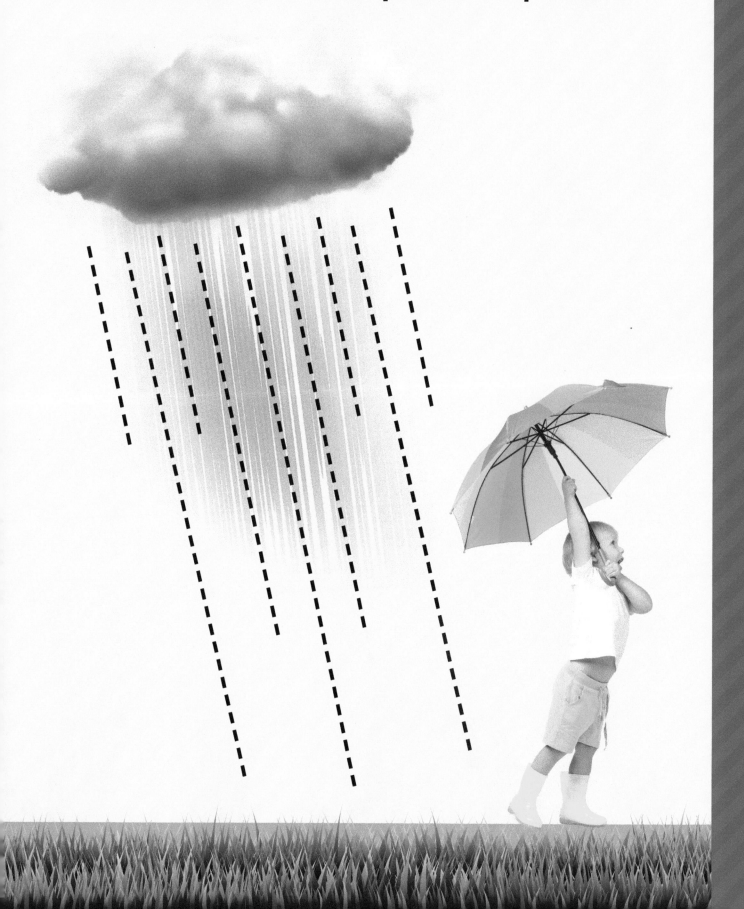

Trace the dotted lines from each number to the matching number of fingers.

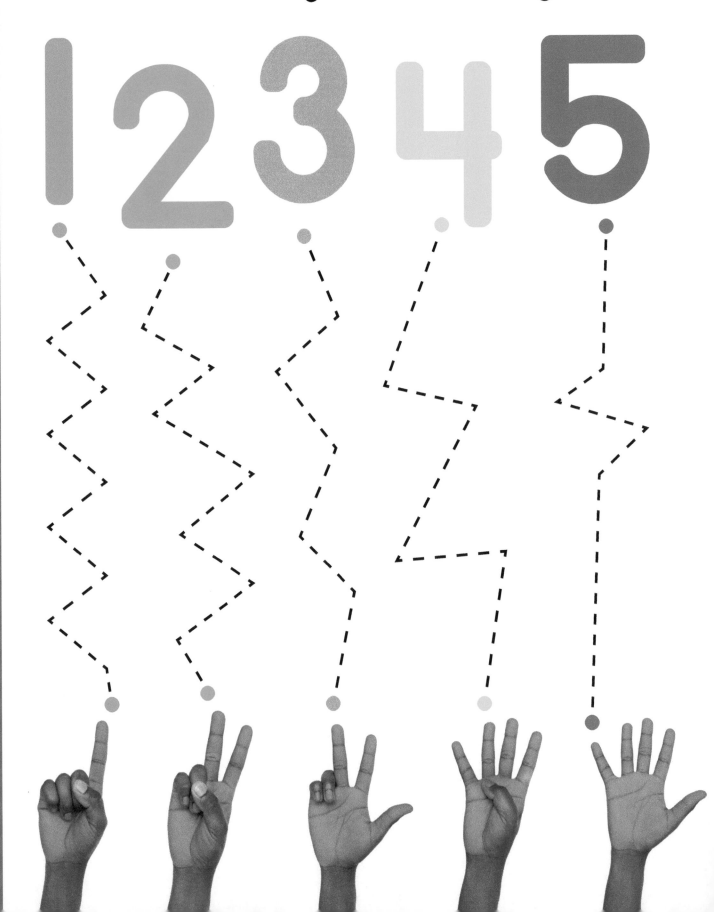

Trace the dotted lines from each dinosaur to its footprint.

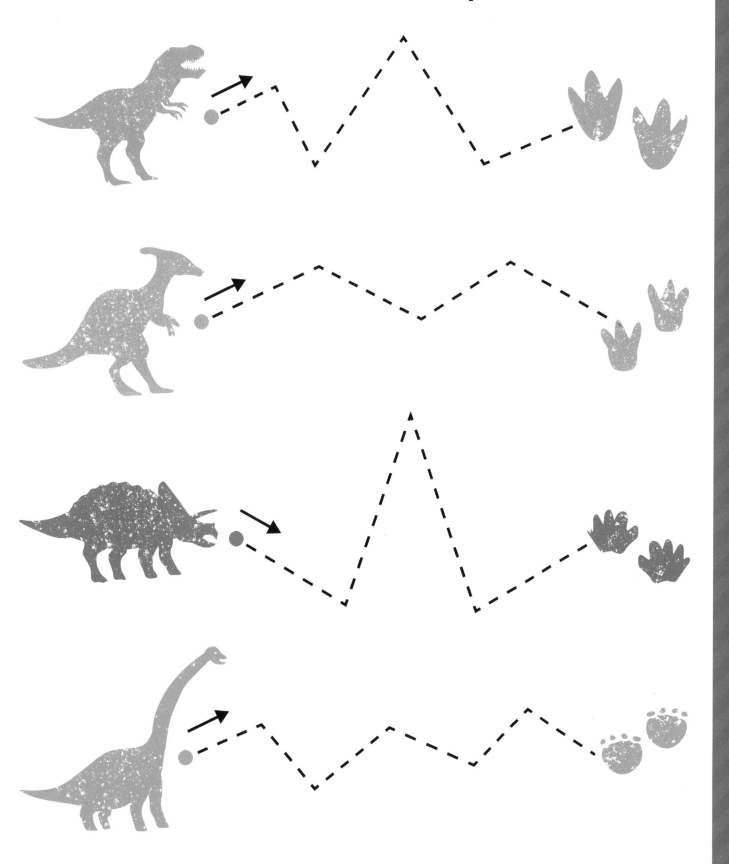

Help the fish swim in the waves by tracing the curvy lines.

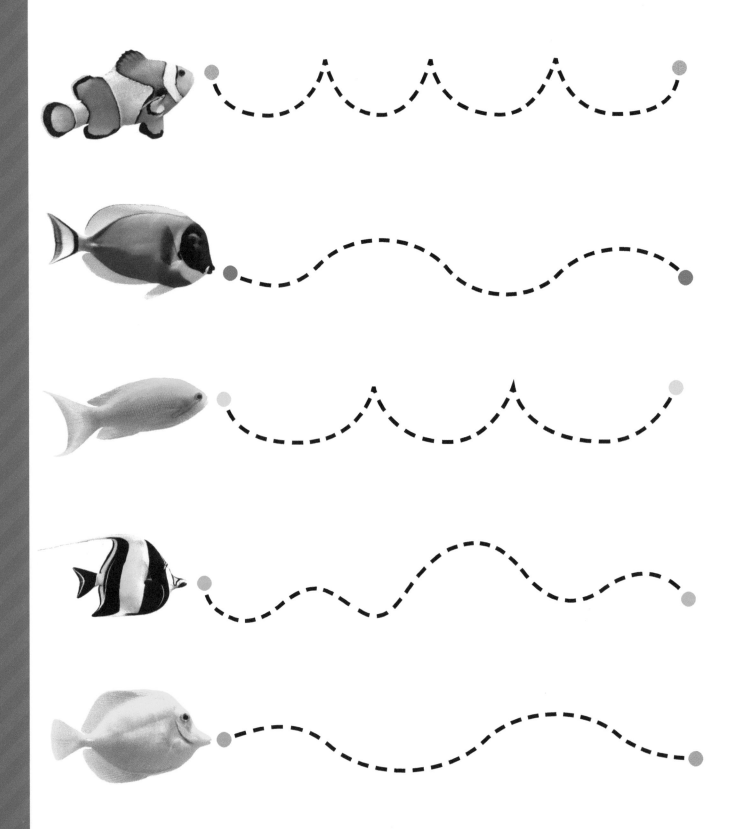

Find the treasure by tracing the dotted lines on the map. X marks the spot!

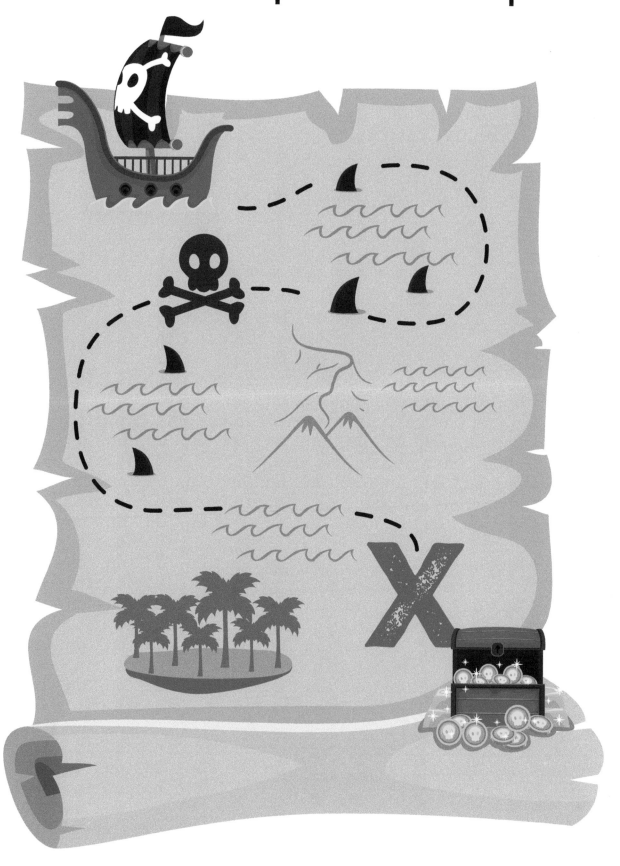

Trace each shape to make a rocket. Then color the picture. 3, 2, 1, blast off!

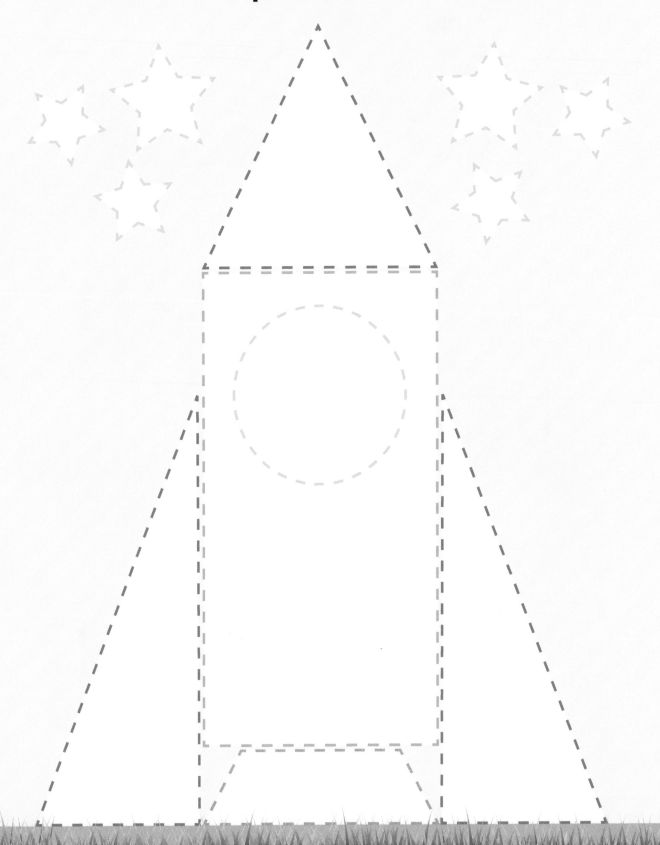

Trace the dotted lines to complete the picture of the umbrella. Then color your picture.

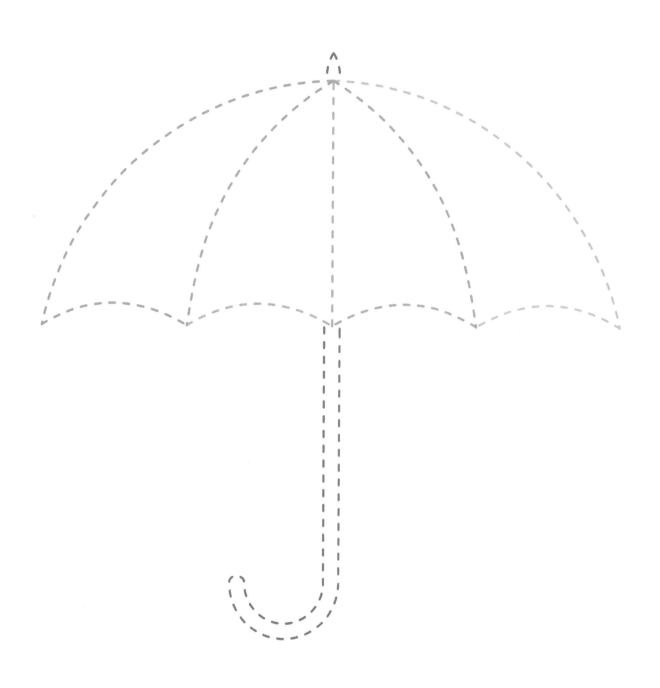

Color the balloons. Try your best to stay in the lines! Then trace the strings.

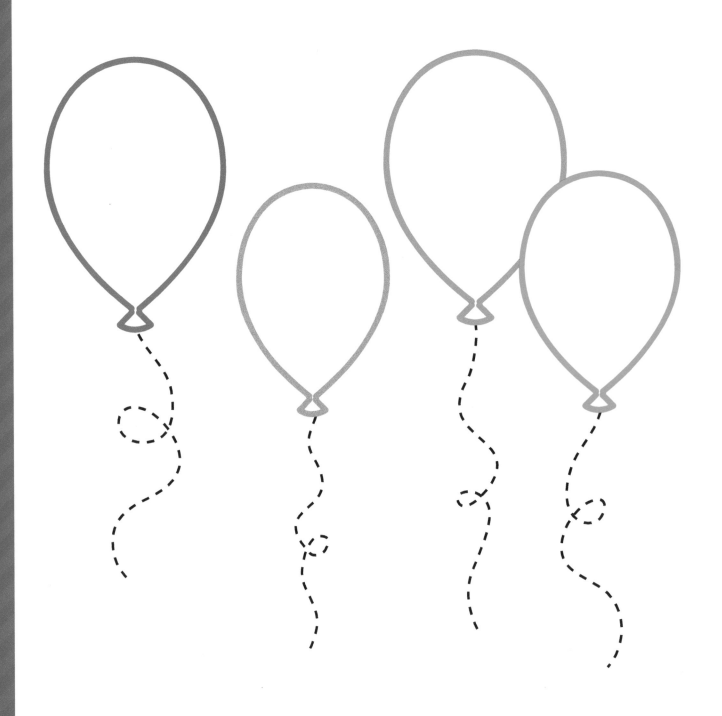

Color the butterfly. Try your best to stay in the lines. How many colors did you use?

Trace the dotted lines to help the animals finish the race. Which one do you think hops the fastest?

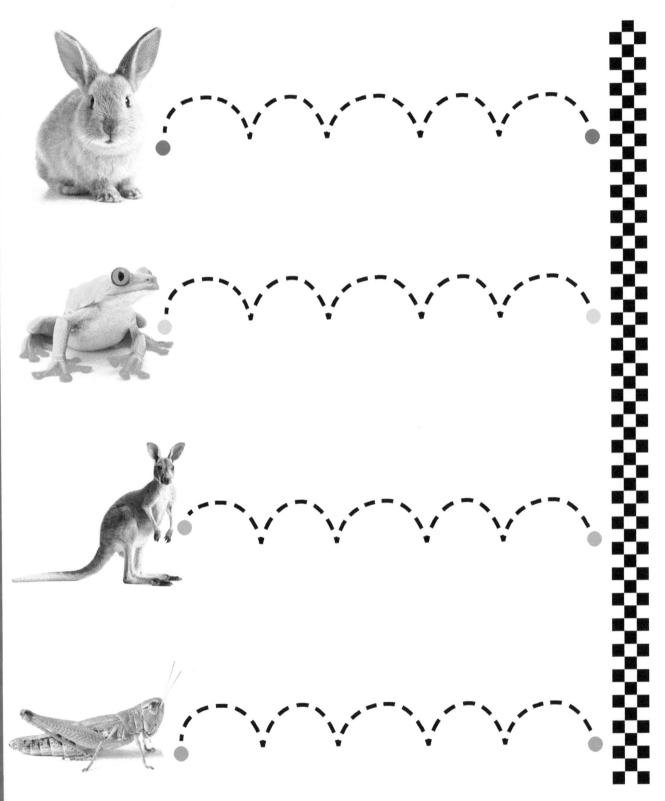

Trace the dotted lines to make the ocean waves. Then color your picture. Try your best to stay in the lines.

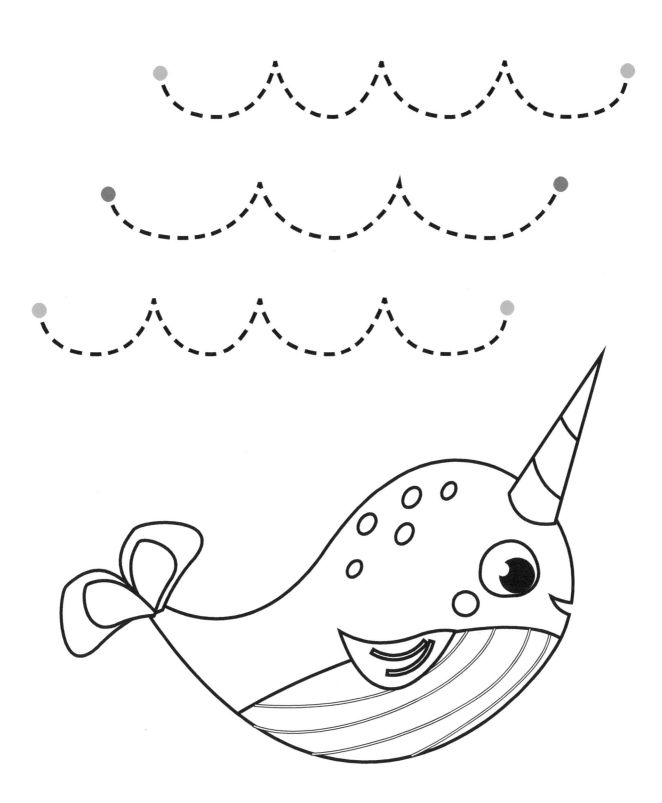

Match the colors by tracing the dotted lines. Can you name each color?

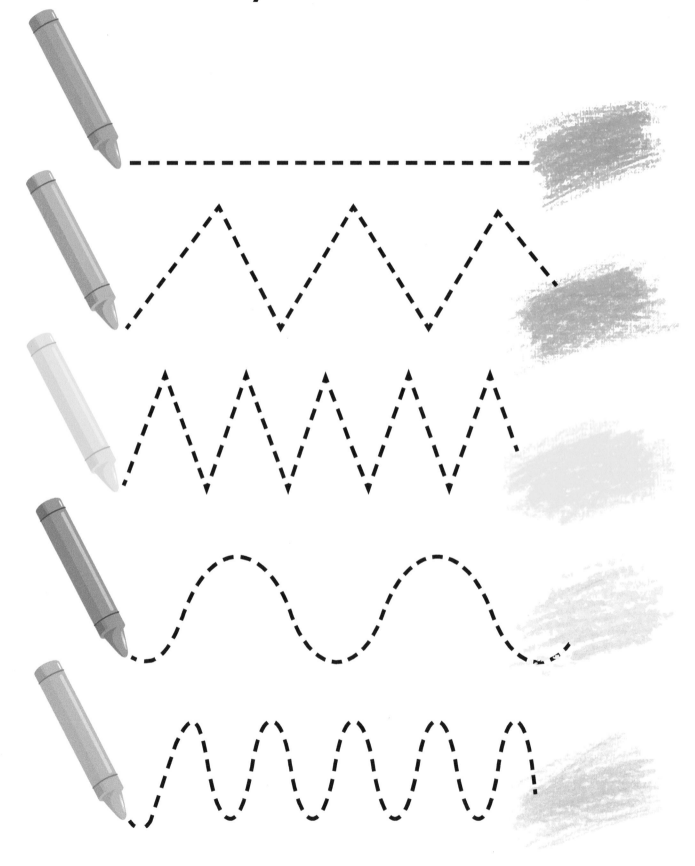

Number Tracing Activities

●▲■▼●●■●▲■▼●●■●▲■▼●●■●▲■

DIRECTIONS

Your little one is ready to start writing! In this section, they will trace numbers and number names. They will also have space to practice freehand all by themselves. Remind them to follow the directional arrows at the beginning of each number and letter. They should focus on staying on the dotted line to correctly form each number. While they are tracing, take the time to say the name of the number aloud and count the corresponding number of objects on the page. This will help your little writer better understand the number. Celebrate their efforts along the way, because writing is a difficult skill to master.

You will also find review activities and games throughout this section. These allow your child to revisit what they have learned as the numbers increase in complexity. It is also an opportunity to practice counting while they take a fun break.

Happy writing!

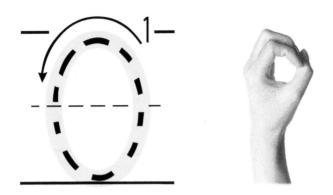

Trace each number. Start at the 1. Pay attention to the arrows.

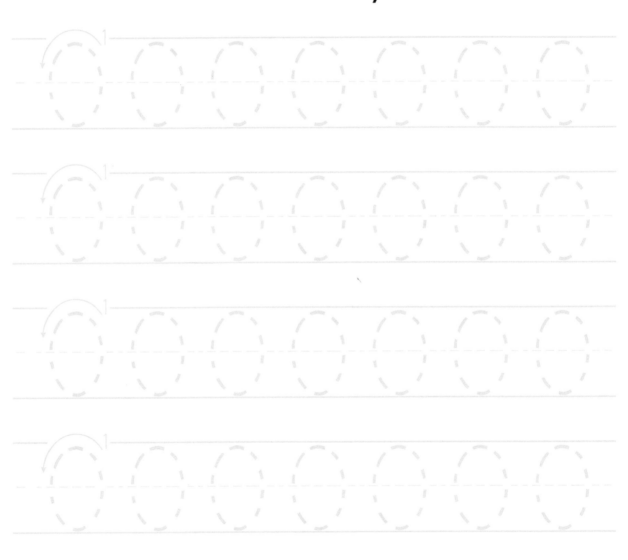

Now, write the number.

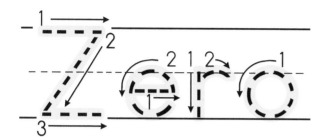

Trace each word. Start at the 1. Pay attention to the arrows.

Now, write the word.

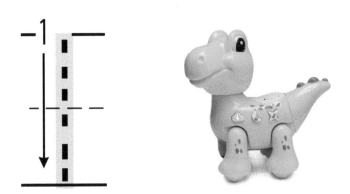

Trace each number. Start at the 1. Pay attention to the arrows.

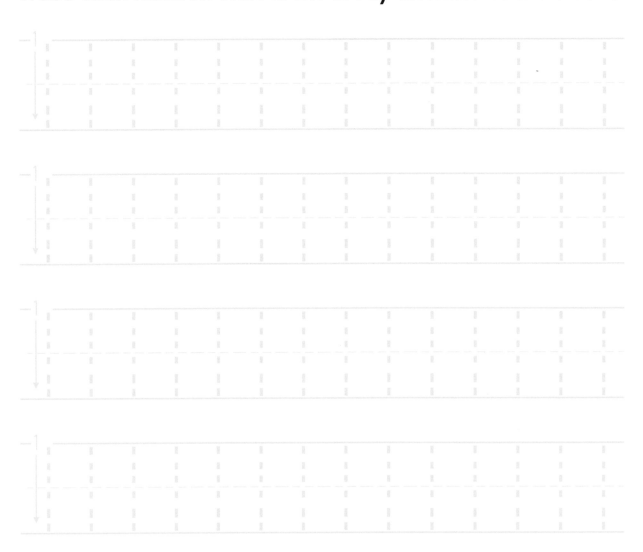

Now, write the number.

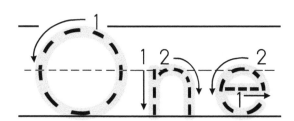

Trace each word. Start at the 1. Pay attention to the arrows.

Now, write the word.

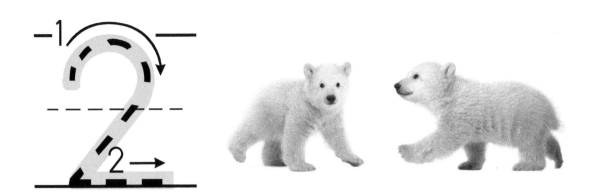

Trace each number. Start at the 1. Pay attention to the arrows.

Now, write the number.

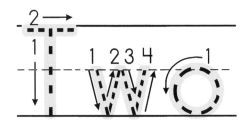

Trace each word. Start at the 1. Pay attention to the arrows.

Now, write the word.

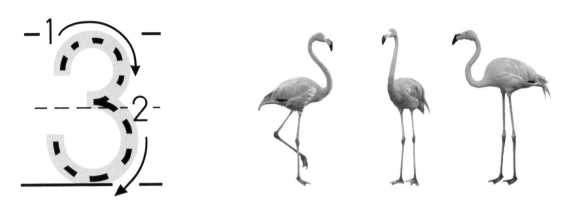

Trace each number. Start at the 1. Pay attention to the arrows.

Now, write the number.

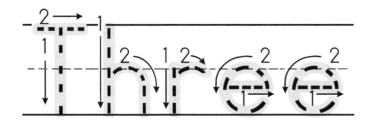

Trace each word. Start at the 1. Pay attention to the arrows.

Now, write the word.

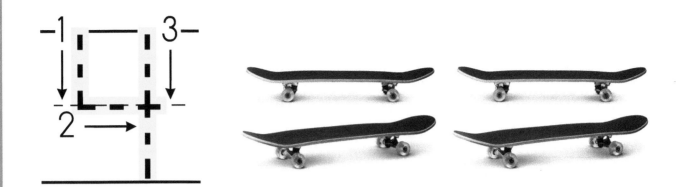

Trace each number. Start at the 1. Pay attention to the arrows.

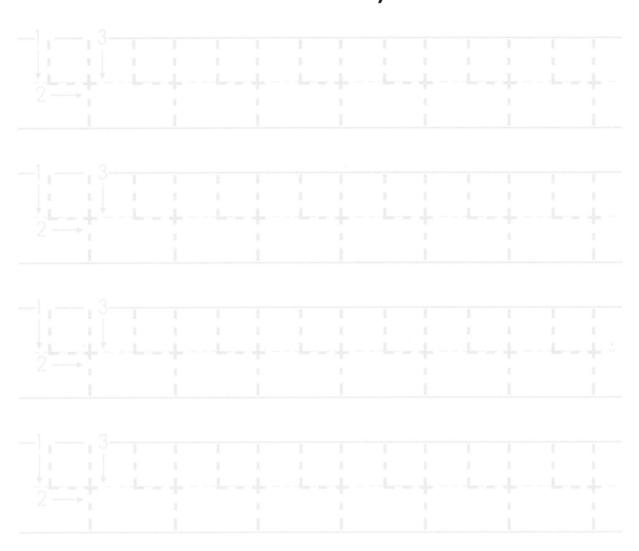

Now, write the number.

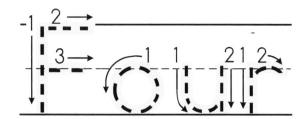

Trace each word. Start at the 1. Pay attention to the arrows.

Now, write the word.

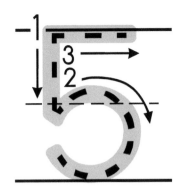

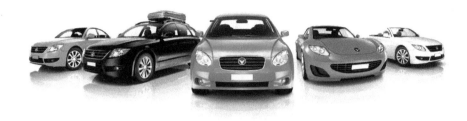

Trace each number. Start at the 1. Pay attention to the arrows.

Now, write the number.

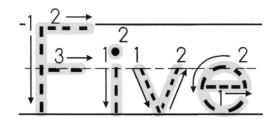

Trace each word. Start at the 1. Pay attention to the arrows.

Now, write the word.

Count the blocks in each stack.
Then trace each number.

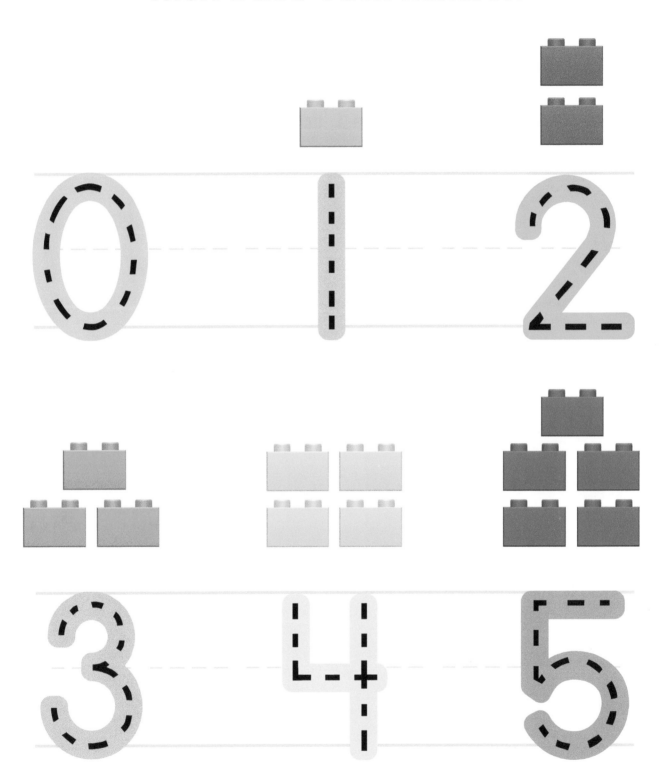

Follow the path of numbers through the maze. Trace each number. How many animals do you see at the zoo?

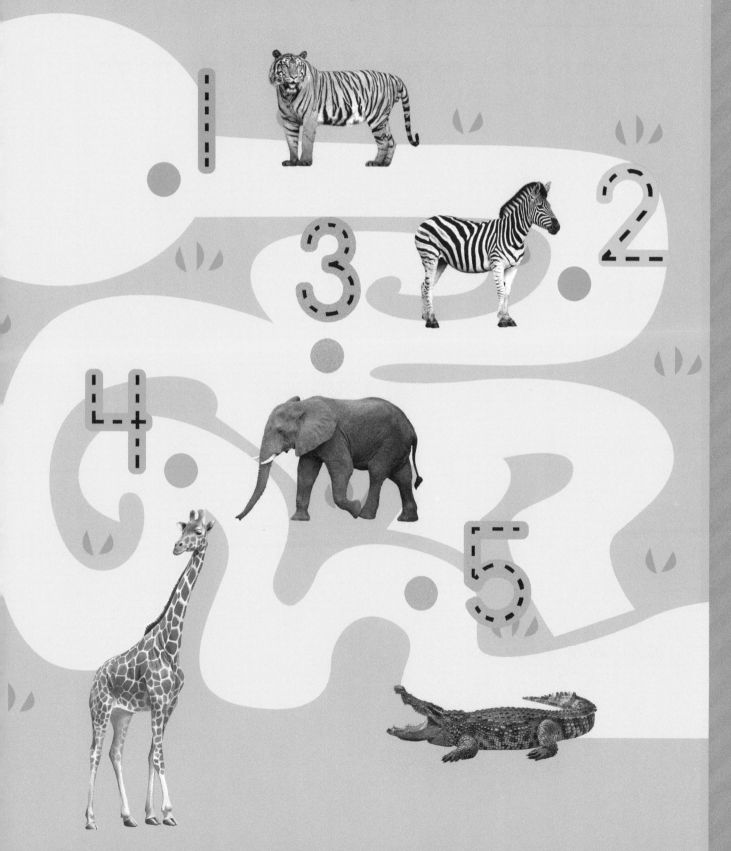

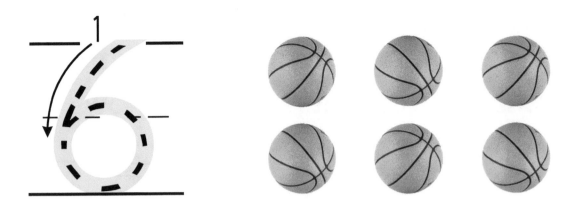

Trace each number. Start at the 1. Pay attention to the arrows.

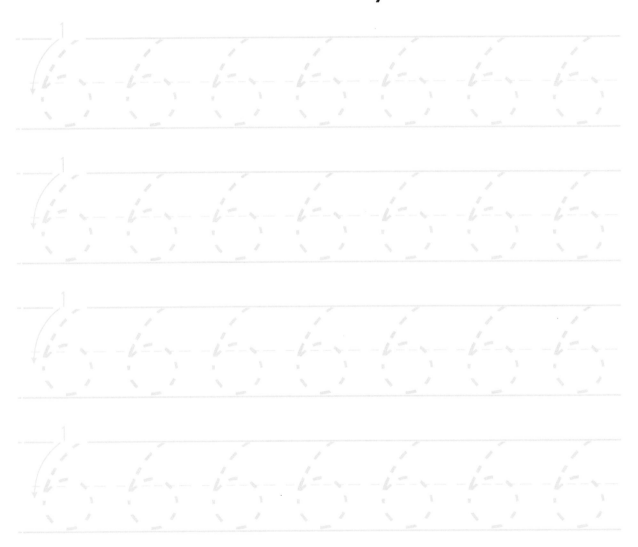

Now, write the number.

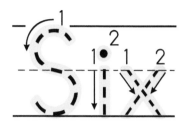

Trace each word. Start at the 1. Pay attention to the arrows.

Now, write the word.

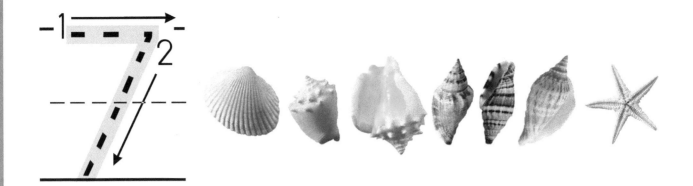

Trace each number. Start at the 1. Pay attention to the arrows.

Now, write the number.

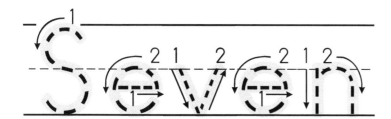

Trace each word. Start at the 1. Pay attention to the arrows.

Seven

Seven

Seven

Seven

Now, write the word.

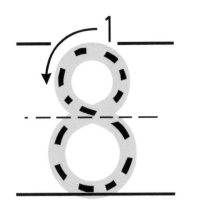

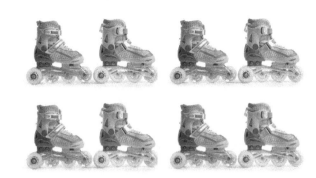

Trace each number. Start at the 1. Pay attention to the arrows.

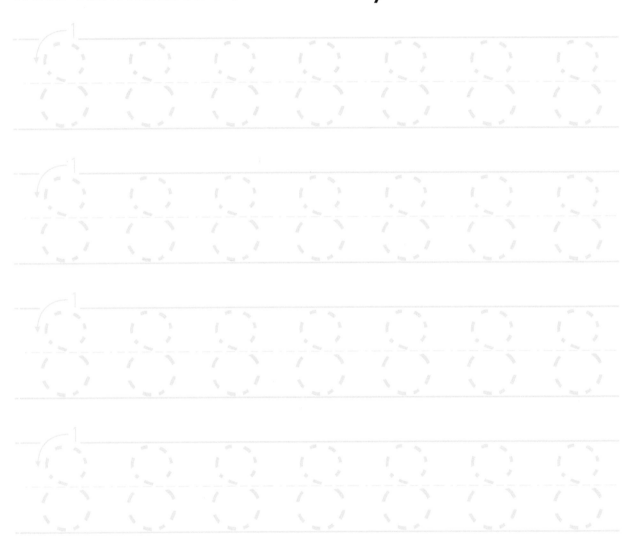

Now, write the number.

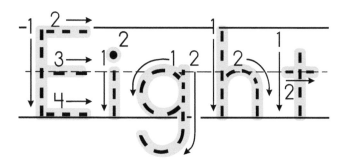

Trace each word. Start at the 1. Pay attention to the arrows.

Now, write the word.

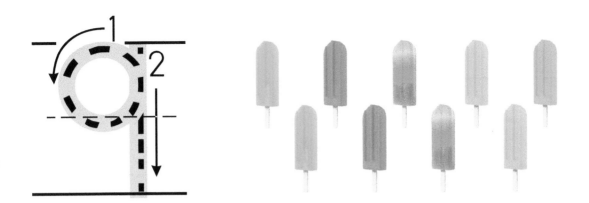

Trace each number. Start at the 1. Pay attention to the arrows.

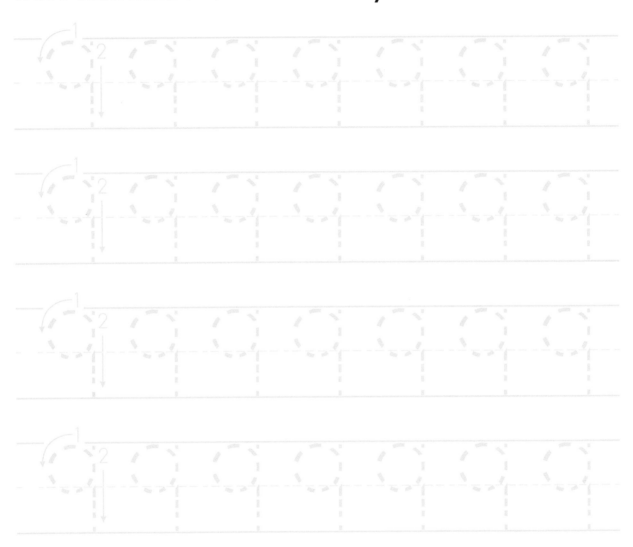

Now, write the number.

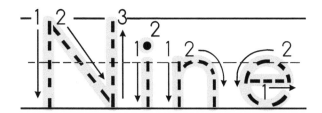

Trace each word. Start at the 1. Pay attention to the arrows.

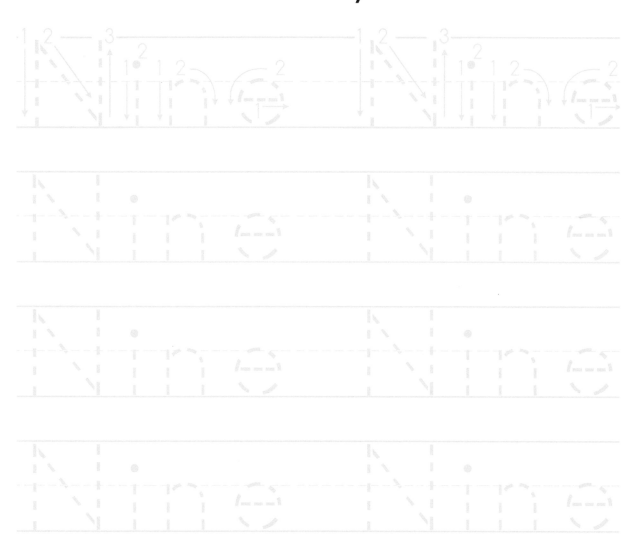

Now, write the word.

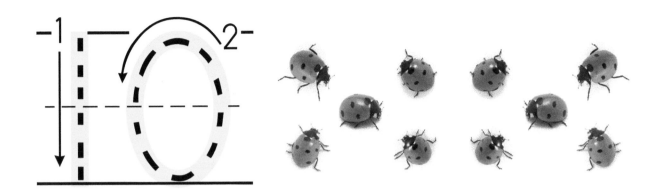

Trace each number. Start at the 1. Pay attention to the arrows.

Now, write the number.

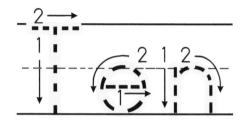

Trace each word. Start at the 1. Pay attention to the arrows.

Now, write the word.

Trace the numbers on the flowers.
How many flowers do you see?

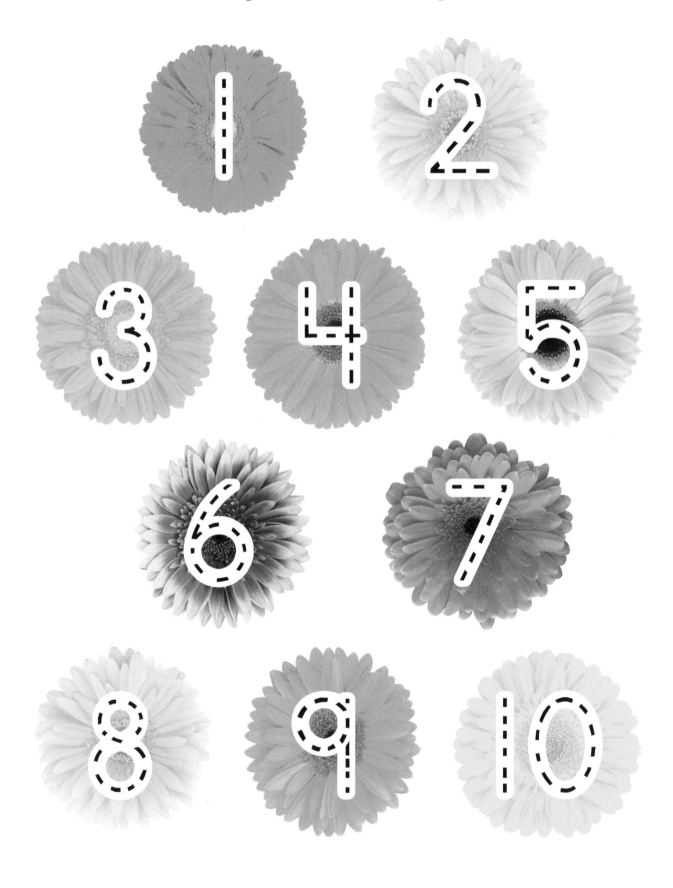

Help the mouse get the cheese. Follow the numbers 1 to 10 in order. Trace each number and count as you go.

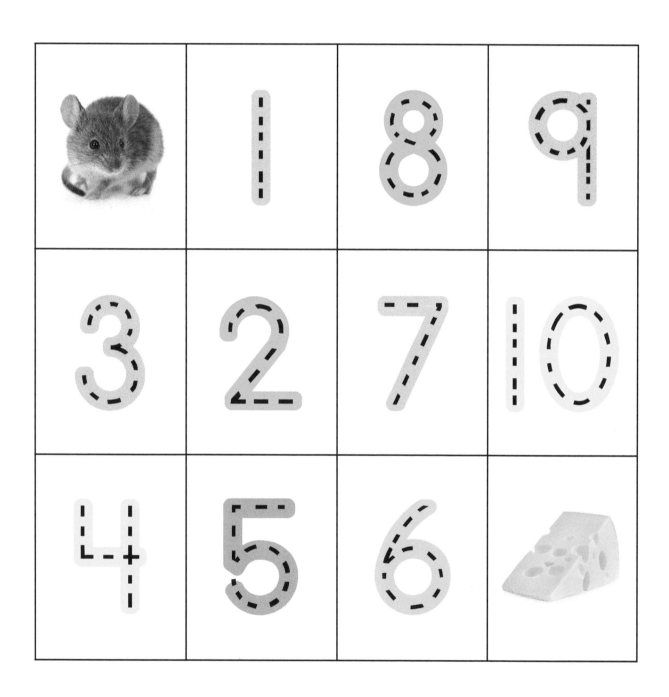

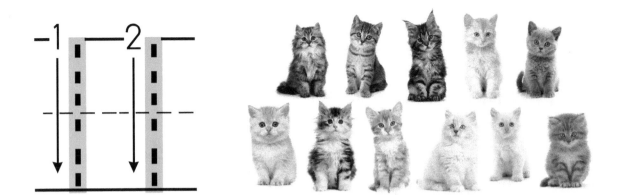

Trace each number. Start at the 1. Pay attention to the arrows.

Now, write the number.

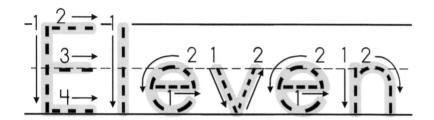

Trace each word. Start at the 1. Pay attention to the arrows.

Eleven

Eleven

Eleven

Eleven

Now, write the word.

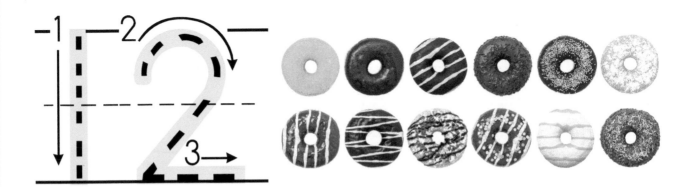

Trace each number. Start at the 1. Pay attention to the arrows.

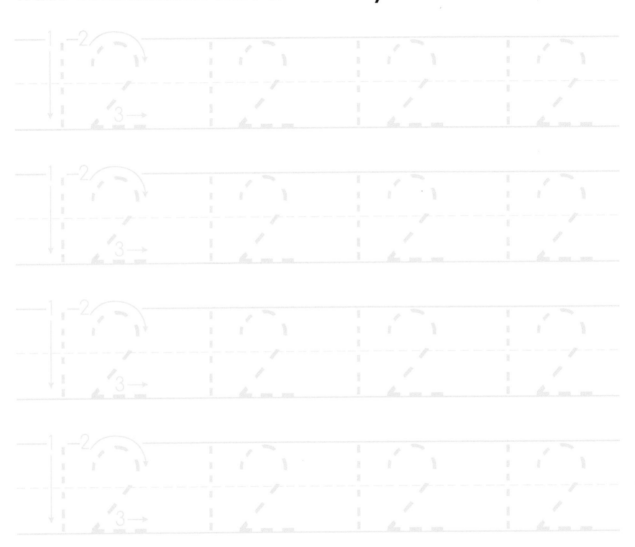

Now, write the number.

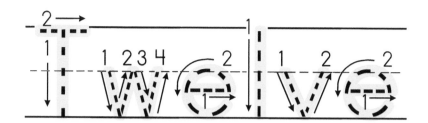

Trace each word. Start at the 1. Pay attention to the arrows.

Now, write the word.

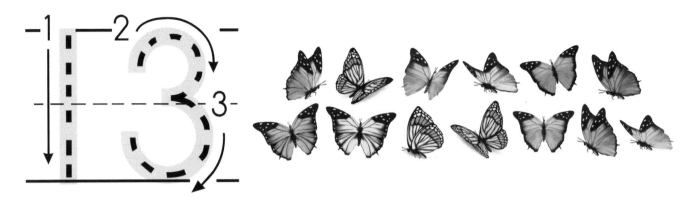

Trace each number. Start at the 1. Pay attention to the arrows.

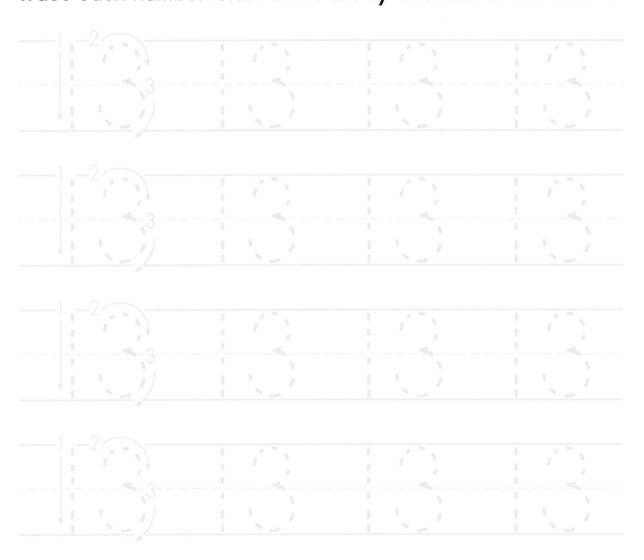

Now, write the number.

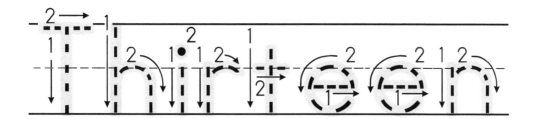

Trace each word. Start at the 1. Pay attention to the arrows.

Now, write the word.

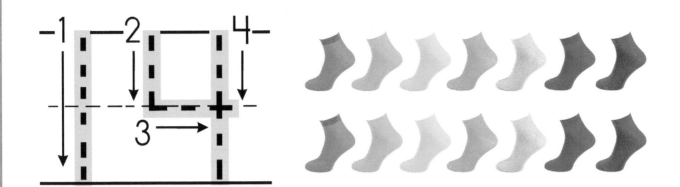

Trace each number. Start at the 1. Pay attention to the arrows.

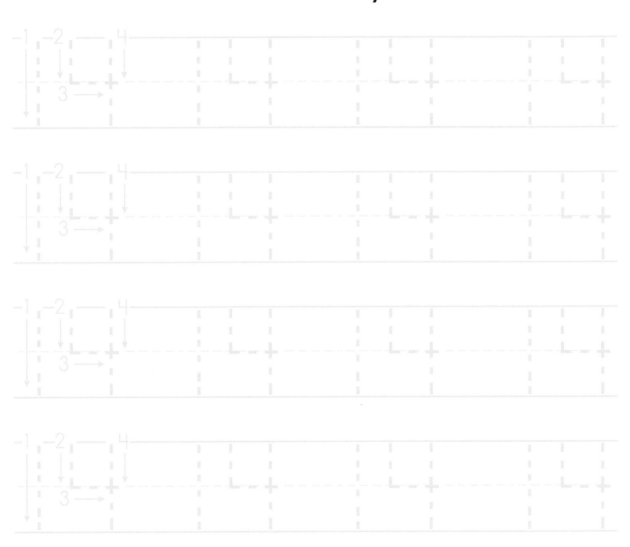

Now, write the number.

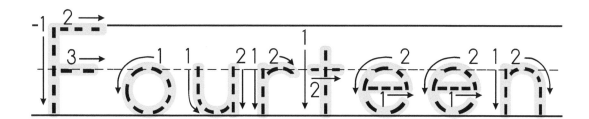

Trace each word. Start at the 1. Pay attention to the arrows.

Fourteen

Fourteen

Fourteen

Fourteen

Now, write the word.

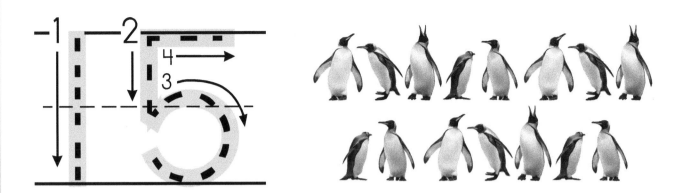

Trace each number. Start at the 1. Pay attention to the arrows.

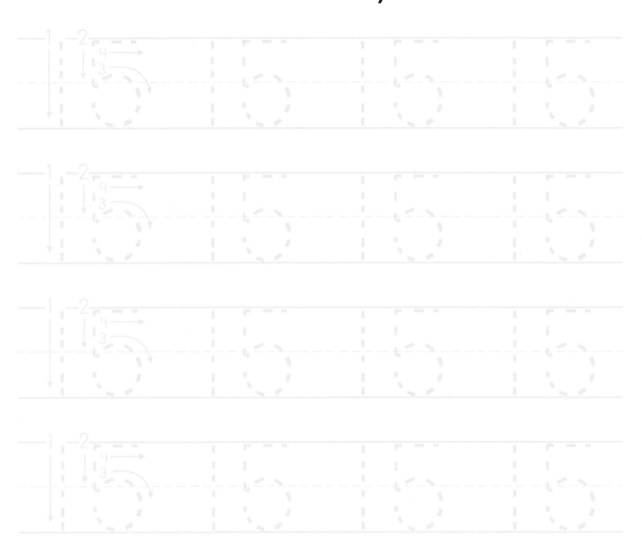

Now, write the number.

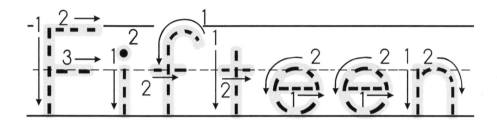

Trace each word. Start at the 1. Pay attention to the arrows.

Now, write the word.

Trace the number on each cupcake.
How many cupcakes do you see?

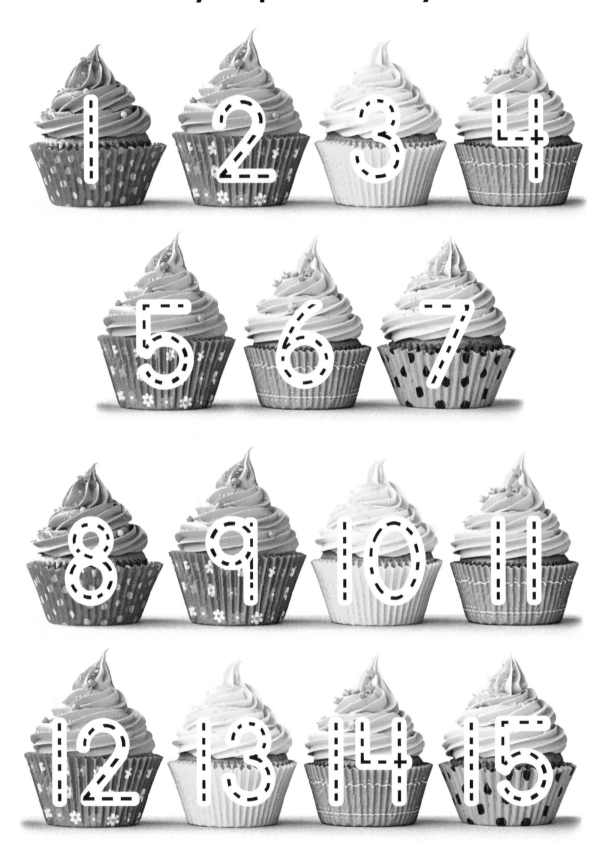

Ride the motorcycle through the maze!
Trace a line through the numbers in order from 1 to 15.

	1	2	9
15	4	3	7
6	5	12	13
7	10	11	14
8	9	5	15
11	3	6	

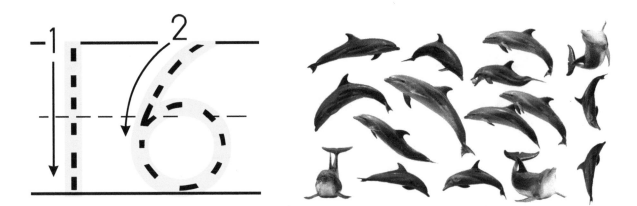

Trace each number. Start at the 1. Pay attention to the arrows.

Now, write the number.

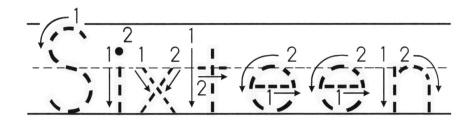

Trace each word. Start at the 1. Pay attention to the arrows.

Sixteen

Sixteen

Sixteen

Sixteen

Now, write the word.

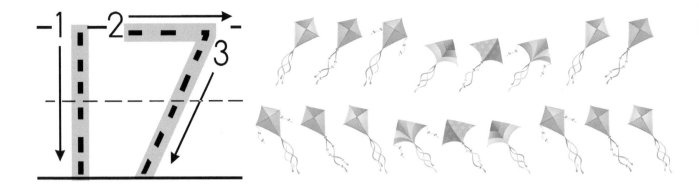

Trace each number. Start at the 1. Pay attention to the arrows.

Now, write the number.

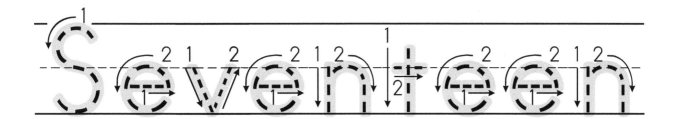

Trace each word. Start at the 1. Pay attention to the arrows.

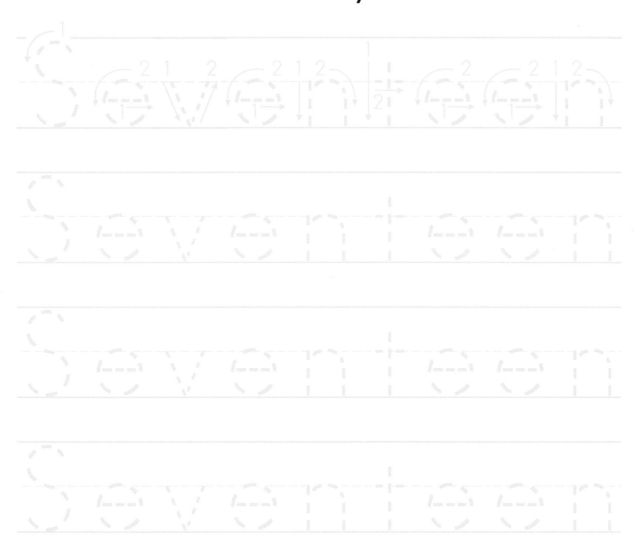

Now, write the word.

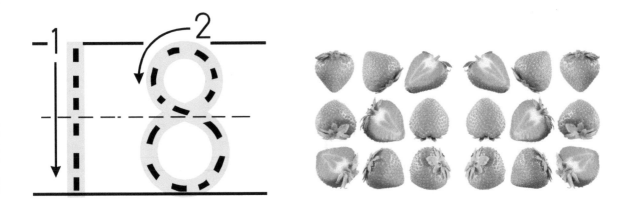

Trace each number. Start at the 1. Pay attention to the arrows.

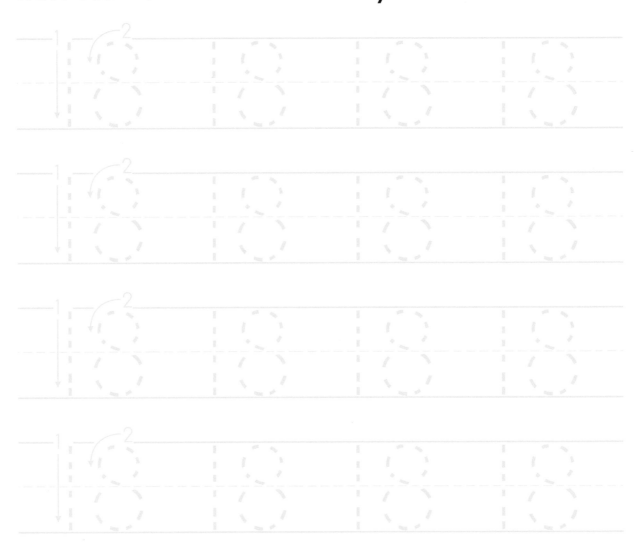

Now, write the number.

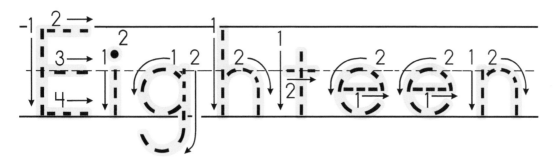

Trace each word. Start at the 1. Pay attention to the arrows.

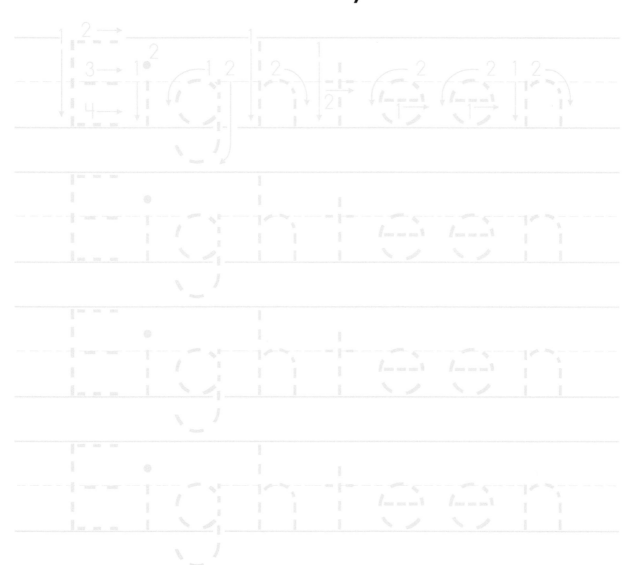

Now, write the word.

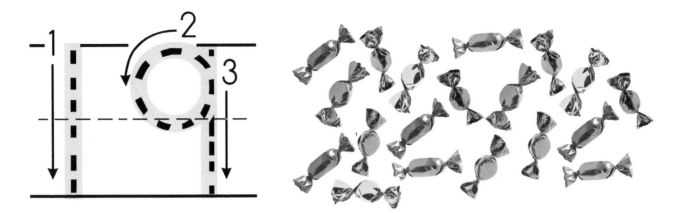

Trace each number. Start at the 1. Pay attention to the arrows.

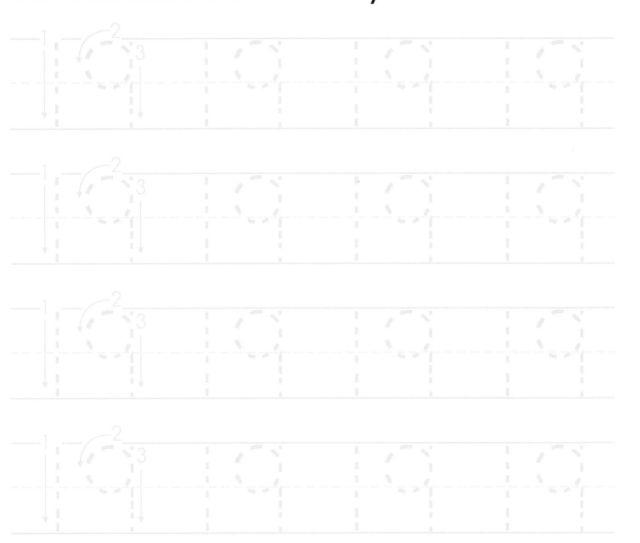

Now, write the number.

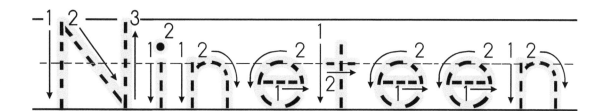

Trace each word. Start at the 1. Pay attention to the arrows.

Now, write the word.

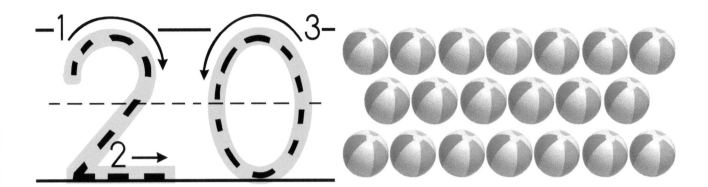

Trace each number. Start at the **1**. Pay attention to the arrows.

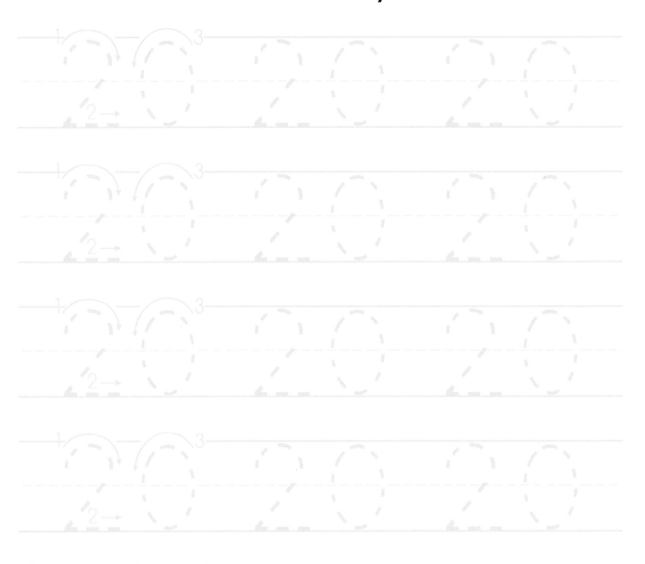

Now, write the number.

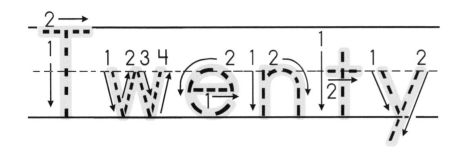

Trace each word. Start at the 1. Pay attention to the arrows.

Now, write the word.

Trace the numbers that the animals are holding.

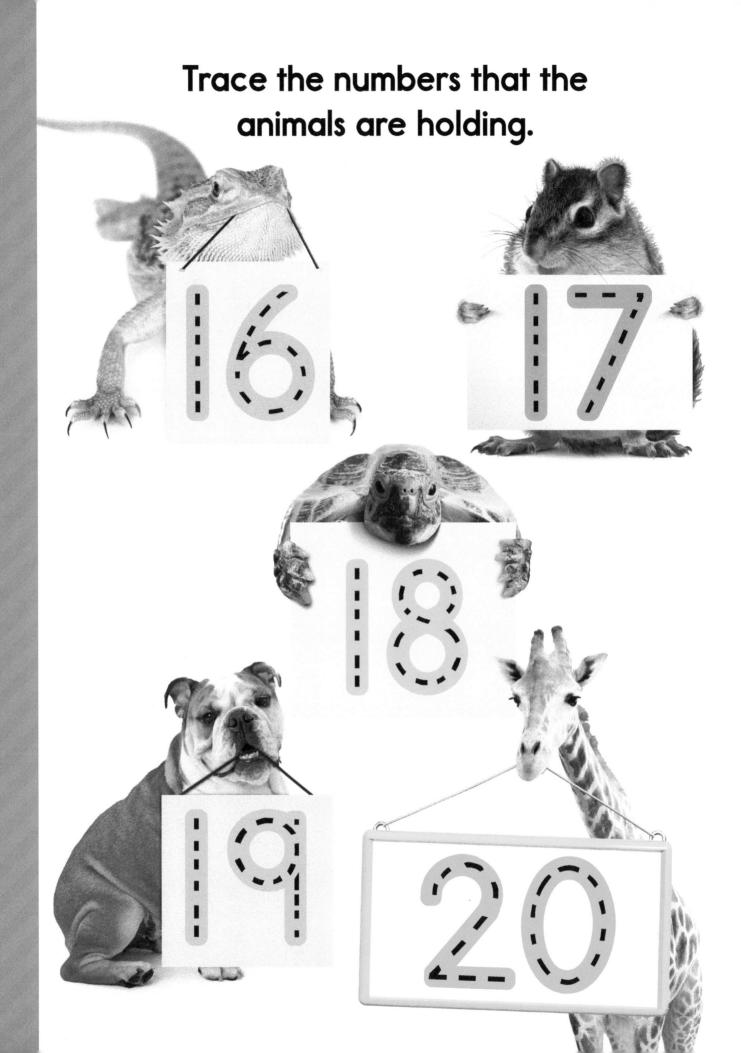

Trace the numbers in the correct order to help the train arrive at the station.

1		5	6
2	3	4	7
5	12	11	8
14	13	10	9
15	16	19	20
8	17	18	Station >

Trace each number. Then count the foods.

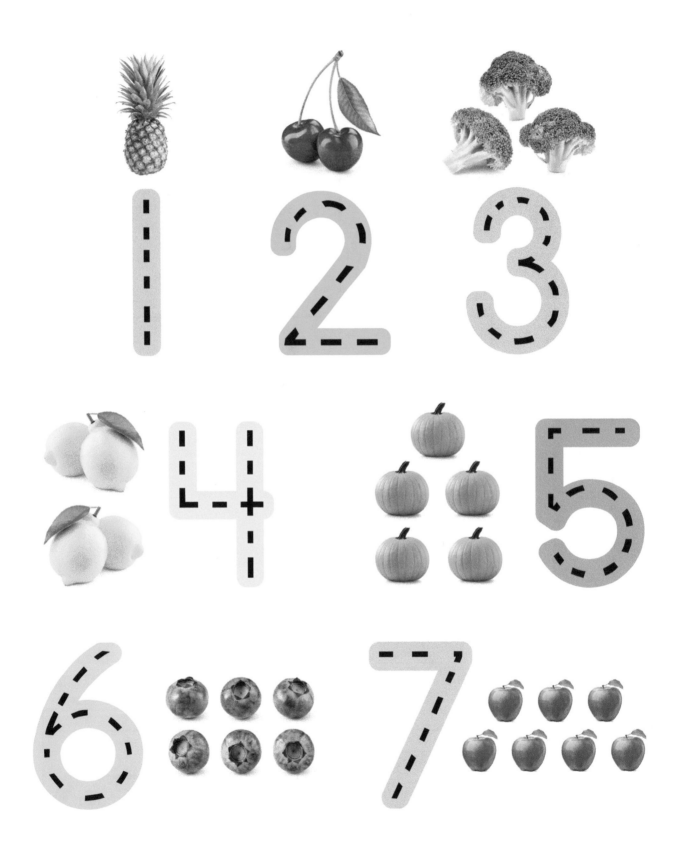

8

9

10

11

12

13

14

15

16

17

18

19

20

This certificate is presented to

for learning to write numbers!

Date _____

About the Author

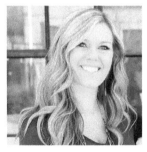

Rachael Smith is the founder and curriculum designer of Literacy with the Littles (LiteracyWithTheLittles.com). Through her blog, she shares crafts and activities for parents and teachers that are designed to help children develop a love of learning. In 2010, she earned her bachelor's degree in Early Childhood Education and began her teaching career. Rachael is a former first-grade teacher turned stay-at-home mom. She is a wife and mother of four little ones. She enjoys crafting, traveling, spending time outdoors, and making memories with her family.

CPSIA information can be obtained
at www.ICGtesting.com
Printed in the USA
BVHW020332021021
617603BV00003B/3